Wheat Free Cookbook

Wheat Free Recipes for a Healthy Wheat Free Diet and Delicious Wheat Free Cooking

Marcia Hansen

Table of Contents

Introduction:

Learning to eat wheat free can be a completely new experience. Whether you have discovered you have a wheat allergy or you just want to eliminate wheat from your diet to enjoy a healthier diet, it can take some getting used to. Wheat free cooking requires some research and learning to cook without ingredients like wheat flour. This wheat free cook book is packed with helpful information on cooking wheat free, a look at some of the benefits of wheat free cooking, some essential tips and tricks to remember and plenty of great wheat free recipes. You will even find some delicious wheat free bread recipes. Eating wheat free does not mean you have to miss out on great tasting food. Use this book as your own go-to resource for changing your life and enjoying delicious, wheat free foods.

Chapter 1: Cooking Wheat Free – What Does it Mean and What are the Benefits?

If you have decided to start eating wheat free or your doctor has recommended a wheat free diet, you may wonder what cooking wheat free really means. Many people mistake a wheat free diet for a gluten free diet. While they do have some similarities, they are not the same. While wheat does have gluten in it, other grains can have gluten as well. This means that wheat free foods may still have gluten in them, which is important for individuals to consider if they need to avoid both wheat and gluten. If you are just avoiding wheat and not gluten, you do have some extra options when you change your diet. A wheat free diet includes avoiding anything that contains wheat or wheat by products.

Top Benefits of a Wheat Free Diet

Your doctor may recommend that you go on a wheat free diet, which means this diet will offer you certain benefits. However, even if you do not have a wheat allergy, you still may be able to enjoy some great benefits when giving up wheat and focusing on wheat free cooking. While it definitely takes some work to eliminate all wheat from your diet, you may be surprised at the benefits you enjoy once you embrace this way of eating. The following are several of the top benefits you can enjoy when you go on a wheat free diet.

Benefit #1 – Better Control Blood Glucose Levels

One of the main benefits you can enjoy when embracing a wheat free diet is the benefit of better control over your blood glucose levels. Wheat is a big contributor to the levels of blood sugar in your body. When you begin eliminating wheat from your diet, you can enjoy lower blood glucose levels. This can help to prevent other diseases like obesity, gluten intolerance and even obesity. It is especially helpful to those who are already suffering from diabetes, since cooking wheat free can help better control blood sugar without the use of insulin or other diabetes medications.

Benefit #2 – Improve Overall Body Health

Another benefit of eating a wheat free diet is the benefit of improving your overall health. When you cut out wheat from your diet, you lower your blood sugar levels, helping to curb cravings for sweets. This not only curbs sweet cravings, but it can help you reduce your appetite as well while eating healthier food choices. Making these changes helps to improve overall health and can help reduce blood pressure, cholesterol levels and more.

Benefit #3 – Enjoy Better Digestion

Many people that eat wheat products have digestive problems, such as water retention, bloating, gas and other digestive discomfort. Wheat can be difficult to digest, which makes intestines work harder. Sometimes blockages or sluggish digestion can occur. When you begin engaging in wheat free cooking, you may notice that you enjoy better digestion. Your digestive system gets a break, which means you may no longer deal with water retention, bloating and gas anymore.

Benefit #4 – Help Lose Weight or Avoid Weight Gain

Going on a wheat free diet may also help you lose weight or may help you to avoid weight gain in the future. Many people find that eliminating wheat from their diet helps to jump start their weight loss plan. Simply try going without wheat products for a couple weeks and you may be stunned with the difference. When you eliminate wheat products from your diet, you will eliminate refined carbs like breads, crackers, cookies and pastas. This can help you to lose weight and once you reach your goal weight, eating a wheat free diet can help you avoid gaining that weight back in the future.

Benefit #5 – Avoid Ending Up with Celiac Disease

Eliminating wheat from your diet may have the benefit of helping you to avoid ending up with Celiac disease. You could have a wheat intolerance and not be aware of it. In fact, studies actually show that Celiac disease is very underdiagnosed today. Consider going on a wheat free diet for a few weeks, even if you do not currently have Celiac disease. You may notice that you feel a lot better without the wheat products in your diet. This could be a sign that you have a wheat intolerance and going off wheat products now can help you avoid further problems like Celiac disease.

Chapter 2: Wheat Free Cooking Tips and Tricks

More and more people today are deciding to go with a wheat free lifestyle. Since many people suffer from gluten sensitivities, Celiac disease and wheat intolerance, it is easy to see why this style of cooking has become so popular. Some even decide to go with wheat free cooking because they simply find it a healthier lifestyle. Getting started with a wheat free diet can be a bit tricky, but with a few tips and tricks, you can be well on your way to cooking many delicious wheat free recipes. The following are some great cooking tips and tricks you can use as you begin your wheat free life.

Be Aware of Ingredients that Contain Wheat
When you take on the wheat free lifestyle, one of the most important things you must do is begin being aware of ingredients that contain wheat in them. While you probably know that most pastas, breads and cakes include wheat in them unless they are specifically labeled "wheat free" or "gluten free," you may not be aware of other commonly used ingredients that have wheat in them as well.

When preparing meals that are wheat free, you will also need to avoid ingredients like most instant chocolate drink mixes, salad dressing mixes and prepared baking mixes. Most gravy mixes include wheat in them as well. Meats that contain fillers, such as sausages and hot dogs often have wheat in them. Other ingredients that contain wheat include malt vinegar, soy sauce, cream soups and Worcestershire sauce.

Great Substitutions to Use for Wheat Free Cooking
The good news is that you can easily find many great substitutions that can be used for wheat free recipes. The following are a few of the general substitutions used for wheat free cooking:

- Barley
- Rice
- Quinoa
- Organic puffed rice
- Pure buckwheat
- Steel cut oats
- Jerusalem artichoke
- Rice flour based bread and baking mixes
- Corn – including corn pasta, corn tortillas, corn starch and corn crackers
- Amaranth

- Millet, puffed millet and millet flour
- Rice noodles
- Sprouted rye rolls and breads
- Parsnips
- Potatoes
- Ground flaxseeds
- Sorghum
- Arrowroot powder
- Chick peas
- Tapioca
- Cornmeal or tortilla crumbs
- Wheat free tamari

Here are some popular substitutions you can use in place of a cup of wheat flour when converting recipes to wheat free recipes on your own:

- 5/8 cup of potato starch flour
- 1 cup of finely milled corn flour
- ½ cup of potato starch flour and a ½ cup of soy flour
- 7/8 cup white or brown rice flour
- ¼ cup of potato starch flour and 1 cup of soy flour
- 1/3 cup of rice flour, 1/3 cup of soy flour and 1/3 cup of potato flour

Some recipes require some kind of thickener and wheat flour is often used in these recipes. Instead of using the wheat flour, here are some substitutions for wheat flour when using it as a thickener within a recipe. Any one of the following can be used in place of 1 tablespoon of wheat flour:

- 1 ½ teaspoon of potato starch
- 1 ½ teaspoon of gelatin
- 1 ½ teaspoon of cornstarch
- 1 tablespoons of white or brown rice flour
- 2 teaspoons of quick-cooking tapioca flour
- 1 ½ teaspoons of sweet rice flour
- 1 ½ teaspoons of sago palm starch
- 1 ½ teaspoons of arrowroot starch

Using Wheat Free Ingredients – Tips and Suggestions
As you begin experimenting with wheat free recipes and using substitutions, you will find that non wheat options perform a bit different within recipes. Here are a few helpful tips and suggestions to use as you begin your journey into wheat free cooking.

- When using oat flour, it offers a nice chewiness to your baked goods but it can be quite sticky.

- You will notice that non-wheat flours are quite a bit heavier in their texture, which means they usually will take about three times as much leavening as you would originally need if using wheat flour.

- Rice flour and barley flour are both quite heavy but they taste a lot like wheat flour. They work well when used in combination with other types of flour.

- When using soy flour, you should only use small amounts of it because it is quite heavy.

- Potato flour and tapioca flour both offer great holding power and work well in recipes that need good holding power. Sometimes you can add them to other non-wheat flours to make sure the recipe sticks together when it needs to.

- Cornmeal or corn flour is more crumbly than wheat flour, which means you usually need to use it along with another type of flour instead of on its own to ensure your recipe will stick together correctly.

Chapter 3: Wheat Free Bread Recipes

If you are dealing with a wheat allergy or you have decided to eliminate wheat from your diet, you may quickly find that you miss eating bread from time to time. The good news is that you do not have to give up bread if you decide to pursue wheat free cooking. It is possible to purchase wheat free bread products and you can also try your hand at making your own wheat free bread, which is often more cost effective. Although bread without wheat may not have the same exact texture and taste you are used to, you will find some excellent wheat free bread recipes that are very tasty. From delicious rolls, to loaves of bread and other bread products, here are some wonderful recipes that you can try to start enjoying bread again while cooking wheat free.

Easy Honey Sweetened Wheat-Free Bread Recipe

Even if you have never tried making bread before, this simple recipe is easy to make and tastes delicious with the added honey and apple.

What You'll Need:

2 teaspoons of active dried yeast
1 ¼ cups of warm water
2 tablespoons of honey (more or less to personal taste)
1 egg
1 apple (the kind of apple doesn't matter), peeled and then finely grated
1 ½ cups of rolled oats
1 ½ cups of brown rice flour (or white rice flour)
2 tablespoons of olive oil
1 egg
½ teaspoon of salt (optional)

How to Make It:

In a large mixing bowl, dissolve the honey in the warm water. Once honey is dissolved, sprinkle yeast on the surface of the water. Allow yeast to sit for 10-15 minutes until it has a frothy appearance on the surface. As the yeast is sitting, take the time to gather the rest of your ingredients together and peel and grate your apple.

Once the yeast has the frothy look on top, add all ingredients and stir together thoroughly. The dough will be wet and does not need to be kneaded.

Bread can be baked in several ways. It can be baked as one large loaf or it can be baked in smaller muffins. Before adding dough to muffin tins or loaf tins, grease the tins thoroughly. Put dough into muffin or loaf tins and allow to rise in a warm area until nearly doubled.

Once the dough is done rising, preheat the oven to 400 degrees F. For muffins, only bake for 25-30 minutes. For bread loaves, bake for 40-45 minutes. Check bread in the last 10 minutes to avoid overbrowning the top.

Simple Soda Bread

This is a heavier bread that tastes delicious, especially when warm. Serve it up with butter, spread with cream cheese, or even add cheese to the tasty warmth of the bread when it comes out of the oven. It is also wonderful with peanut butter or jam. Since it is heavier, it can be used to make bruschetta or for dipping in soups. No yeast is used with this bread, so you have no rising time to worry about.

What You'll Need:

2 cups of rice flour
1 ¾ tablespoons of softened margarine
1 teaspoon of cream of tartar, heaped
1 level teaspoon of baking soda
1 egg, beaten
1 cup of buttermilk
Pinch of salt

How to Make It:

Preheat the oven to 400F
Use a large mixing bowl and combine together the rice flower, cream of tartar, salt and baking soda together.

Rub in the margarine with the dry ingredients, rubbing well until you have no lumps left. In a smaller bowl, whisk the beaten egg and buttermilk together. In the large bowl, create a well in the middle of the ingredients, pouring the liquid into the well. Use your hands to begin mixing the dry and wet ingredients together. Mix well with hands to get the dough to hold together.

Turn out the dough on a floured surface, kneading gently for two minutes. Shape into a round loaf about 5-6 inches in diameter, placing onto a greased baking sheet. Use a knife to make a cross cut on the loaf that is about halfway through the loaf. Bake at 400F for 30-40 minutes, checking during the last 10 minutes for desired doneness.

Remove from the oven and the remove from the baking sheet, placing on a wire rack to cool. Serve warm for the best taste and texture.

Wheat-Free Savory Wheat Free Bread Recipe

For a tasty savory addition to any meal, this wheat free bread recipe is a winner. It bakes up to be a wholesome, delicious bread that tastes wonderful warm and when cool. Try toasting leftovers for a savory snack or breakfast with a bit of butter. The Savory Wheat-Free Bread from Wheatfree-Bread-Recipes.Blogspot.com inspired this recipe.

What You'll Need:

1 cup of warm vegetable water (water used to steam vegetables)
1-2 teaspoons of honey
1 tablespoon of active dried yeast
½ teaspoon of dried herbs of choice, like parsley (or you can use a tablespoon of fresh herbs)
½ onion, chopped finely
1 apple, any kind, peeled and then finely grated
1 cup of rolled oats
¼ cup of ground almonds
1 cup of brown rice flour
¼ cup of quinoa flakes
2 tablespoons of olive oil

1 large egg

½ teaspoon of salt (optional)

How to Make It:

Preheat oven to 400F

Use a large mixing bowl and place warm vegetable water in the bowl, then dissolving the honey into the warm water. Sprinkle yeast on top of the water and allow to set for 10-15 minutes or until the yeast has become frothy on top.

While you are waiting on the yeast, chop the onion, peel the apple, grate the apple and then gather all the needed ingredients together. Once the yeast has become nice and frothy, add all ingredients to the mixing bowl, stirring very thoroughly until you have a nice, wet batter. This batter will be very wet and does not need to be kneaded. If the batter seems too wet to get into a muffin tin or a loaf tin, add just a little bit more of the brown rice flour.

This bread recipe can be made into muffins or you can make it into a nice loaf. Make sure you grease the pans before adding the dough. Place dough in muffin or loaf pans, allowing to rise until close to doubled in size in a warm place. Bake for 30 minutes at 400F.

Rosemary Spiced Wheat Free Flat Bread Recipe

This is another savory bread recipe and since it is a flat bread, it uses no yeast. It is best eaten the same day it is made and is especially tasty when warm. It is a wonderful compliment to soups or just a nice snack to enjoy. The rosemary gives it a savory flavor. You can experiment with the amount of rosemary used in the recipe to get the flavor that best suits your taste.

What You'll Need:

1 ½ teaspoon of granular yeast

1 ¼ cup of warm water (approximately 100 degrees and avoid making it too hot or you will kill the yeast)

1 ½ cup of brown rice flour

2 teaspoons of sugar (or substitute in honey if you are avoiding sugar)

1 tablespoon of olive oil

4 egg whites at room temperature

4 teaspoons of dried rosemary or 6-8 teaspoons of fresh rosemary

12 black oils cured in oil, pitted and chopped roughly

1 garlic clove (large), peeled and then cut into 2-4 pieces

1 egg yolk combined with a ½ teaspoon of water

½ cup of cornstarch

1 teaspoon of salt

2 teaspoons of xanthan gum powder

½ cup of corn flour

How to Make It:

Begin with glass two-cup measuring cup, stirring the yeast, ½ cup of the warm water, brown rice flour and sugar together. Allow to sit in a warm area for about 10-15 minutes until it has doubled in volume.

Meanwhile, take a large baking sheet and line it with parchment paper. Use a 8 inch cake pan and trace two 8-inch circles onto the parchment paper.

In a small bowl, lightly beat the egg whites. Then, add two teaspoons of the rosemary (3-4 teaspoons if using fresh), chopping olives and olive oil. Sit this to the side.

In another small bowl, combine the egg yolk mixture with the garlic and sit to the side, allowing the garlic to add flavor to the glaze without allowing the garlic to burn.

Combine together the corn flour, rice flour, salt, cornstarch and xanthan gum powder within a large mixing bowl. Add the leftover ¾ cup of warm water to the olive oil and egg white mixture, then stirring this into the dry ingredients. Next, stir in your doubled yeast mixture. Beat these ingredients into you have a nice, smooth dough. The dough should be soft and smooth.

Use a rubber spatula to spread dough into the circles that you marked out on your parchment paper. Allow dough to heap up in the middle of the circle. Lightly spray or grease a long amount of plastic wrap, using it to cover the loaves of bread. Place in a warm area and allow to rise for about an hour, or until the bread dough has doubled in size.

Preheat the oven to 425F. Take the garlic out of the glaze mixture and then brush the egg yolk glaze on top of both loaves. Use the leftover rosemary to sprinkle the tops of the bread loaves. Use a sharp knife or razor blade to create a slashed diamond grid pattern on top of the loaves (this is optional).

Bake at 425F for 20 minutes, ensuring that the tops are nicely browned before removing from the oven. Serve right away or allow to cool on a baking rack.

Wheat Free Bagel Recipe

If you enjoy having a bagel for breakfast now and then, you may be wondering how to still enjoy this delicious treat while eating wheat free. This wheat free bagel recipe tastes great. Simply toast bagels up and eat with cream cheese or other toppings. While this recipe takes a few steps and a little work on your part, it's worth it to enjoy those warm bagels. You may want to double or triple the recipe and freeze leftovers to enjoy later. This way you only do the work once and you will have bagels to eat for several weeks.

What You'll Need:

½ cup of tapioca flour
2/3 cup of rice flour
1 ¾ teaspoon of xanthan gum
1 tablespoon of sugar and 1 teaspoon of sugar, divided
2 tablespoons of dry milk powder
1 teaspoon of salt
1 tablespoon of dried yeast
½ cup of warm water
2 tablespoons of butter or margarine
2 egg whites
¼ cup of hot water

Extra sugar to coat bagels
Extra rice flour

How to Make It:

Start by placing dry milk powder, tapioca flour, rice flour, 1 tablespoon sugar, xanthan gum and salt into a food processor or mixer. In the ¼ cup of hot water, place the butter or margarine and dissolve it, stirring to make sure it completely combines.

In a bowl, place the ½ cup of warm water, stirring in the 1 teaspoon of sugar until it is completely dissolved. Then, sprinkle dried yeast on the top of the water, allowing to sit for about 10 minutes until it is foamy and frothy.

In the mixer or food processor, blend together the dry ingredients on low. Add the dissolved butter or margarine with water to the mix, mixing once again on low until well combined. Add in the yeast mixture and the egg whites, mixing again on low until thoroughly mixed. You should have a thick dough that should hold its shape. If it is not thick enough, add a bit more of the rice flour, mixing again and then checking out the dough's consistency. If your dough is too thick, you can add a small amount of water, adding until you have the dough to the right consistency.

Now, put the mixer on high, beating the dough for 4-5 minutes. You may need to use dough hooks if you have them.

Line baking sheets with some parchment paper or you can spray them with cooking spray, then dusting with a bit of the rice flour.

Divide the dough into eight equal sections. Make sure you keep hands floured with rice flour or grease them. Rolle each portion into a ball. Flatten the ball slightly, poking a hole into the center, making it large enough so it will not close while baking. Your dough should now have a nice bagel shape.

Place bagels on prepared baking sheets, covering with sprayed or greased plastic. Allow bagels to sit in a warm area for about 30-60 minutes, or until the bagels have doubled in size.

To get that great shiny, crispy coating that bagels have, bring a large saucepan of water to a rolling boil, adding a teaspoon of sugar to the water and allowing it to totally dissolve. Once dissolved, drop bagels into the boiling water, one by one, allowing to cook for 30 seconds, then turning and cooking for 30 seconds on the other side. Remove carefully with a slotted spoon, placing the bagel back on the baking sheet.

Preheat oven to 400F. Bake the bagels at 400F for 20-22 minutes, checking to make sure they do not get too brown in the oven. They taste best when still slightly warm, but they will still be great for the next couple days. Freeze them if you will not be eating them within 3-4 days of baking them.

Wheat Free Dinner Rolls Recipe

What You'll Need:

1/3 cup of corn flour
1/3 cup of rice flour
½ cup of tapioca flour
1 teaspoon of xanthan gum
1 tablespoon of potato flour
1 ½ teaspoon of baking powder
1 teaspoon of unflavored vegetarian gelatin
1 ½ tablespoons of sugar, divided
½ teaspoon of salt
2 ¼ teaspoons of dry yeast granules
1 cup of warm water
1 egg, beaten
1 teaspoon of vinegar
2 tablespoons of olive oil or canola oil

How to Make It:

Preheat the oven to 375F.

Place lightly oiled baking rings on a baking pan.

In a large mixing bowl, mix together the corn flour, rice

flour, tapioca flour, xanthan gum, potato flour, salt, baking powder and gelatin. Set to the side.

In glass 2-cup measuring cup, add warm water and then dissolve a teaspoon of sugar into the water. Sprinkle the yeast on top of the warm water, allowing to sit until it becomes foamy.

In a small mixing bowl, mix together vinegar, oil, egg and the remaining sugar. Add the yeast mixture to this bowl and combine. Then, pour the liquid ingredients into a well that is made right in the middle of the dry ingredients. Mix together very well. Beat until smooth with a large wooden spoon, which should only take a few minutes.

Spoon batter into the baking rings (rings are needed to keep the batter from spreading too much). Cover the baking sheet with greased plastic, allowing the rolls to rise until they have nearly doubled. This takes 30-45 minutes.

Bake for 20-22 minutes at 375F. Avoid allowing the rolls to get too dark. Once you take the rolls out of the oven, remove the rings right away and move rolls to a wire rack where they can cool. This keeps rolls from getting soggy. Makes six rolls. For more rolls, you can always double the recipe. Serve up while they are still warm with butter or jam.

Wheat Free Sorghum Flax Bread

This is one of the healthiest wheat free bread recipes you will find, since it is fully of healthy goodness, including ingredients like flaxseed. The addition of maple syrup adds a touch of sweetness to this wheat free bread and it slices up nicely. Eat it toasted for breakfast or add it to any meal on the side. This recipe was inspired and adapted from Laurie Sadowski's recipe from "The Allergy-Free Cook Bakes Bread: Gluten Free, Dairy Free, Egg Free."

What You'll Need:

2 ½ teaspoons of active dry yeast
1 ½ cups of warm water and 1 tablespoon of warm water, divided
2 tablespoons of pure maple syrup (or you can use agave nectar)
½ cup of potato starch
¼ cup of bean flour
¼ cup of ground flaxseeds and 3 tablespoons of flaxseeds, divided
½ cup of quinoa flour
¼ cup of tapioca flour
¾ cup of sorghum flour and 2 tablespoons of sorghum

flour

1 teaspoons of sea salt

2 ½ teaspoons of xanthan gum

2 teaspoons of cider vinegar

2 tablespoons of olive oil or canola oil

How to Make It:

Preheat your oven to 350F. Then oil a loaf pan that measures 8 ½ x 4 ½ inches.

In a large, glass measuring cup, place one cup of the warm water. Stir yeast and maple syrup into the water. Allow to stand for 5-10 minutes or until the yeast has turned foamy. It should have about a half inch of foam on top.

The remaining ½ cup and tablespoon of warm water should go into a large mixing bowl that can be used with a large mixer or a hand mixer. Stir in the three tablespoons of the flaxseeds, allowing to stand until it has thickened up, which takes about 5-7 minutes.

In a medium bowl, combine together the remaining flaxseeds, potato starch, bean flour, tapioca flour, quinoa flour, sorghum flour, salt, and xanthan gum.

Once the water and flaxseed mixture has thickened, add in the vinegar and oil. Mix with a mixer on medium speed for 30 seconds, making sure it is well combined. While continuing to mix on low, begin to add in the yeast mixture gradually. Then slowly add the flour mixture, slowing mixing to make a dough. Turn the mixer off and use a spatula to scrape the sides of the bowl, then go back to mixing for five minutes on medium-high speed. You will end up with a sticky dough.

With your rubber spatula, scrape the dough into the prepared loaf pan. Make sure the top is nice and smooth. Place in a warm area, allowing it to rise while uncovered for about an hour or until the dough reaches the loaf pan's top. Make sure the oven is preheated while the dough is rising.

Bake the loaf for 40-45 minutes. The top should brown nicely and you should be able to insert a toothpick into the loaf's center with it coming out clean if the loaf is completely done. Remove from the oven and then tip the loaf out onto a baking rack to let it cool. Allow it to completely cool before you try to slice it.

Chapter 4: Wheat Free Main Course Recipes

Sometimes wheat free cooking can be a bit of a challenge, especially when you are coming up with main course ideas. This wheat free cook book chapter offers you some excellent main course recipes for delicious wheat free dinners that will not make you feel deprived. All these wheat free recipes are healthy, wholesome and tasty. You can use these wheat free foods for your main course at dinner or for your main course at lunch. Have fun adding some wheat free side recipes to the mix, experimenting with combinations that have complimentary flavors that make every meal extra special. Choose a recipe that looks good, gather your ingredients, make the main course and then enjoy trying out the new dish.

Wheat Free Chicken Tikka Masala Recipe

If you love curried chicken but you are always worried about having it when you eat out because you are not sure it is wheat free, this recipe is a great solution. You can have delicious chicken tikka masala and it is completely wheat free. It is easy to make, it is low in fat and calories and you can enjoy a health, delicious meal that satisfies your craving for curry.

What You'll Need:

Marinade Ingredients:

1 inch of ginger root, fresh
1 cup of plain, low fat yogurt
1 tablespoon of coriander leaves, chopped finely
3 cloves of garlic
1 tablespoon of lime juice
Pinch of garam masala
¼ teaspoon of ground turmeric
½ teaspoon of chili powder
Pinch of salt
Chicken Tikka Masala Ingredients:
4 boneless, skinless chicken breasts, cut into 1-inch cubes

1 large onion, chopped

2 tablespoons of olive oil

1 inch of ginger root, fresh and minced finely

4 cloves of fresh garlic, minced

½ teaspoon of chili powder

1 teaspoon of tomato puree

½ teaspoon of ground turmeric

1 teaspoon of ground coriander

½ green pepper, chopped

1 cup of chopped tomatoes

½ red pepper, chopped

How to Make It:

Place diced chicken into the marinade. This is easiest when placing marinade and chicken in a ziplock plastic bag. Ensure chicken is coated well with marinade and allow to marinate in the refrigerator for about 30-45 minutes.

In a large skillet, heat up the olive oil. Sauté the onion until tender. Add ginger and garlic, cooking for another two minutes. Then, stir in coriander, chili and turmeric, mixing together well. Add in the peppers, chopped tomatoes and tomato puree, allowing the mixture to sauté for another 2-3 minutes.

Take chicken out of the marinade while ensuring that some of the marinade stays on the chicken pieces. Place chicken into the pan, mixing chicken up with the other ingredients. Cover the large skillet with a lid, bringing everything to a boil. Once the mixture is boiling, turn down and allow to simmer for about 25 minutes, stirring from time to time.

Make sure chicken is fully cooked. Once done, serve the chicken and sauce over fluffy Basmati rice. To add a nice contrast, serve mango chutney on the side. Makes four servings.

Healthy Wheat Free Pizza Recipe

Many people love pizza, but buying pizza may be out of the question when you have decided to eat a wheat free diet. Most pizza crust does include wheat, but this great pizza recipe allows you to indulge in pizza while still engaging in wheat free cooking. Not only is the crust wheat free, but all the toppings are fairly healthy as well, so you can enjoy an old favorite the healthy way.

What You'll Need:

Pizza Crust Ingredients:
¼ teaspoon of baking soda
¼ teaspoon of sea salt (or regular salt)
1 large egg
1 tablespoon of extra virgin olive oil
1 ½ cups of almond flour (you can experiment substituting in other alternatives to wheat flour, such as brown rice flour)
Pizza Topping Ingredients:
¾ cup low fat mozzarella cheese
¼ - ½ cup organic pizza sauce or homemade pizza sauce
½ cup of sliced mushrooms
½ pound of ground turkey sausage, cooked
4-8 cherry tomatoes, sliced

10 fresh basil leaves

How to Make It:

Preheat the oven to 350F.

Begin making the pizza crust by combining together the baking soda, sea salt, and almond flour in a mixing bowl. In a small bowl, whisk together the egg and olive oil, whisking well until well combined and smooth. Pour olive oil mixture into the dry ingredients, using a wooden spoon to stir them together until you have created a firm ball of pizza dough.

Turn out the mixture onto a greased baking sheet or pizza pan, pressing the dough into a circle about 10 inches in diameter. Lightly flour hands with a bit of rice flour if the dough is a bit sticky.

Spread pizza sauce over the pizza crust, spreading evenly and leaving a ½ inch border around the outside of the pizza crust for easy handling later. Sprinkle mozzarella cheese over the pizza sauce, then sprinkling the pizza with the cooked, ground turkey sausage. Place cherry tomato slices and sliced mushrooms evenly across the pizza.

Bake the pizza at 350F for about 20 minutes or until the cheese is bubbling. Remove pizza from the oven, topping with the fresh basil leaves. Place back in the oven, baking another five minutes. Remove from oven once again, letting the pizza cool for a few minutes before serving while still warm. Makes 2 servings, so you may want to double this recipe if you are feeding a family.

Cheesy Bacon and Broccoli Pasta Dish Recipe

A delicious, warm pasta dish is a comforting meal, but it gets a bit trickier to make when you are only eating wheat free foods. This cheesy pasta dish combines healthy broccoli with a bit of bacon for a wonderful, saucy pasty dish. You will not need any flour to thicken this sauce either. It is a quick and easy recipe that allows you to get dinner on the table quickly as well.

What You'll Need:

½ cup of sliced button mushrooms
1 cup of small broccoli florets
6 slices of bacon, trimmed and chopped into 1 inch pieces
1 ½ cups of milk
1 teaspoon of olive oil
1 teaspoon of wheat free mustard
1 tablespoon of cornstarch
1/3 cup of grated, sharp cheddar cheese
Black pepper to taste
Wheat free pasta for serving

How to Make It:

In a frying pan, heat olive oil and then fry up bacon or turkey rasher pieces for about three minutes. Add in the broccoli and mushrooms, continuing to fry for another 3-5 minutes. Remove skillet from heat.

Mix together two tablespoons of the milk and the cornstarch in a medium saucepan. Add the leftover milk to the mix, stirring to combining and heating over low to medium heat. Stir continuously until your sauce starts to thicken. When sauce starts thickening, add in the cheese and the mustard, continuing to stir until cheese melts into the sauce.

Add the broccoli, mushrooms and bacon into the cheese sauce, cooking a bit longer to ensure everything is thoroughly heated. Sprinkle with ground black pepper to taste. Serve hot over wheat free past. Makes two servings.

Wheat Free Chicken Risotto Recipe
Chicken risotto can be made without using any ingredients that include wheat. This recipe eliminates any wheat and gives you a great main dish recipe that can be made quickly. It is a healthy recipe that is low in fat and includes tasty vegetables to help you make sure you are eating more veggies each day. Add a size of

steamed broccoli for a full meal that takes a short amount of prep time in the kitchen.

What You'll Need:

2-3 boneless, skinless chicken breasts, chopped into 1 inch pieces
1 cup of risotto rice
1 onion, chopped
1 green pepper, chopped
1 red pepper, chopped
10 medium mushrooms, sliced
2 tablespoons of olive oil and 1 tablespoon of olive oil, divided
3 cups of what free vegetable stock
2 teaspoons of dried oregano
¼ cup of parmesan cheese, grated
Ground black pepper to taste

How to Make It:

In a medium saucepan, heat olive oil and add risotto rice to the pan, heating the rice for 2-3 minutes until it begins looking translucent. Next, add in the mushrooms, onions and peppers, cooking for five more minutes. Make sure you avoid browning the rice.

Add vegetable stock to the saucepan, bringing it to a boil. Turn to low and simmer the rice for 25 minutes. If you need to, add some extra boiling water to avoid allowing the rice to dry out while cooking.

Meanwhile, in a skillet, heat a tablespoon of oil, cooking the chicken pieces in the oil until they are lightly browned and cooked through. Once the risotto is done cooking, add in the chicken, black pepper and oregano. Mix until well combined. Serve hot and top with the parmesan cheese. Makes three servings.

Wheat Free Crunchy Baked Haddock

It is always nice to have that crunchy coating on fish, but you may not be sure how to make a nice coating without using something that contains wheat. This recipe allows you to enjoy a deliciously, crunchy topping for your haddock (or any other white fish) without using flour or other ingredients that contain wheat. This recipe is completely wheat free and offers a tasty, low fat way to enjoy your fish with a crunchy coating.

What You'll Need:

4 fillets of haddock or other white fish
1 cup of plain Greek yogurt
1 lemon peel, finely grated
1 lemon, squeezed for the lemon juice
½ teaspoon of olive oil
½ cup of parmesan cheese
2/3 cup of crushed corn tortilla chips
2 teaspoons of dried herbs to taste

How to Make It:

Preheat oven to 350F.

Take a glass or metal oven proof dish, using the olive oil to lightly oil it.

Mix grated lemon peel together with the Greek yogurt. Sprinkle lemon juice over the fish fillets.

In a plastic bag, place the crushed tortilla chips, parmesan cheese and herbs, shaking the bag well until all the ingredients are mixed.

Dip the fish fillets in the Greek yogurt mixture, ensuring all parts of the fish are well coated. Then, dip the fish into the tortilla chip mix, making sure all parts of the fish are well coated. Place fish fillets in oven proof dish, topping with any leftover tortilla chip mix.

Bake at 350F for 30 minutes. Serve hot. Makes four servings.

Wheat Free Sausage Potato Soup

Many soups require some kind of wheat based ingredient for thickening. This tasty soup does not. It is very filling, cheap to make and you can vary the flavor of the soup by using various types of sausage. Of course, to keep the soup low in fat, we have used turkey sausage for this recipe. Keep in mind, if you decide to use another type of sausage, avoid fatty sausages, since they will result in grease on top of your soup unless you brown the sausage and drain it prior to adding it to the soup.

What You'll Need:

5 cups of wheat & gluten free chicken broth (you can make your own to ensure it is wheat free)
1 large onion, peeled and diced
3 medium potatoes, peeled and thinly sliced
½ pound of wheat and gluten free turkey sausage
½ cup of milk
1 teaspoon of flat leaf parsley, finely chopped
½ teaspoon of salt
¼ teaspoon of freshly ground black pepper
Grated parmesan cheese to sprinkle on top when serving

How to Make It:

In a large saucepan, heat the chicken broth. Add in thinly sliced potatoes and chopped onion, cooking for 1-15 minutes at a light boil until potatoes become tender. Using a slotted spoon, remove the onion and potato from the soup, allowing the liquid to remain warm on low heat.

Place the potatoes and onions in a food processor, processing until they become smooth. Add back into the soup, mixing until well combined. This will thicken the soup for you.

TIP - Make sure you clean your food processor right away, since the processed onions and potatoes become very sticky and are tough to clean up if you let it cool.

Add milk into the soup, allowing to simmer for about five minutes. Stir often to make sure soup does not burn or stick to the bottom. Meanwhile, cook up the turkey sausage, browning lightly to ensure it is well cooked. Dry on paper towels to eliminate any grease or fat. Add sausage into the soup. If using sausage links, slice sausage before adding to the soup.

Allow soup to cook on medium low for about 10 more

minutes, continuing to stir regularly. Season with parsley and pepper. Serve hot into warm bowls, sprinkling the grated parmesan cheese on top of the soup to melt. Eat immediately. Makes 4-6 servings.

Wheat Free Cheesy Tuna Oven Bake

Tuna offers some great health benefits and makes a delicious meal when served up with wheat free pasta. This recipe adds in some healthy vegetables to help you add more veggies to your diet. It offers a quick dish that can be prepared beforehand and then popped into the oven just in time for dinner. Try adding different vegetables to the bake to change up the flavors for something new.

What You'll Need:

1 cup of tuna, canned in water and well drained

1 large can (about three cups) of chopped tomatoes

¾ cup of canned sweet corn

1 tablespoon of tomato puree

½ Italian seasoning

1 clove of garlic, minced or pressed

½ cup of milk

¾ cup of low fat, plain Greek yogurt

1 cup of shredded, low fat mozzarella cheese

2/3 dashes of tabasco sauce

Ground black pepper to taste

Wheat free pasta (enough for two people)

How to Make It:

Preheat oven to 400F.

Cook pasta according to instructions and then drain well. Cook pasta al dente, since you will be baking this meal in the oven.

In a medium saucepan, combine garlic, tabasco, herbs, tomato puree and chopped tomatoes, bringing the mix to a boil and then allowing to simmer for about 10 minutes. Allow the mix to cool to avoid curdling the yogurt.

Add milk, sweet corn and yogurt to the tomato mixture, stirring until well mixed.

Stir tuna into the warm pasta, making sure the tuan is well distributed. Add tomato mixture and stir gently until combined, being careful not to break up the pasta. Add the mixture into a greased ovenproof dish. Top with the shredded mozzarella cheese.

Cook at 400F for 30 minutes or until the food is bubbling and golden brown on top. Makes two servings. Goes well with steamed veggies or a nice salad.

Chapter 5: Wheat Free Appetizer Recipes

Whether you are serving guests with wheat allergies or you want to whip up some delicious wheat free appetizers to enjoy anytime, these delicious recipes are sure to be a huge hit. These recipes are easy to make and let you have great appetizers while sticking to your desire to follow a wheat free diet. Make a single batch for the family or double or triple the recipe to serve a crowd.

Oysters with Wheat Free Dipping Sauce

Oysters are a healthy appetizer that offer a great way to get plenty of zinc in your diet. With a delicious wheat free dipping sauce, you will make the oysters a special appetizer to enjoy. If you will be serving these oysters to guests, serve the oysters on a platter lined with crushed ice to keep them nice and cool.

What You'll Need:

24 fresh oysters laid out on half the shell
1 cup of apple cider vinegar
¼ cup of lemon juice
2 cloves of garlic, pressed or minced
1 tablespoon of fresh, flat leaf parsley, chopped
2 tablespoons of green onions, finely sliced
½ teaspoon of sea salt
1 lemon, sliced into slim wedges for decoration

How to Make It:

In a small bowl, mix the vinegar, lemon juice, garlic, green onions and sea salt together. Allow the ingredients to stand for 30 minutes to allow the flavors to combine. A few minutes before you serve the dish, add in the chopped parsley, tasting the sauce to make sure you do not need to add more lemon or other seasonings. When you are pleased with the taste, prepare the oysters to serve.

On a platter lined with crushed ice, arrange your oysters, using the lemon wedges around the platter for decoration. Spoon approximately a teaspoon of the sauce on every oyster or you can serve the sauce on the side and allow people to drizzle the sauce on the oysters themselves when they are ready to eat them. Serves approximately 4-6 people, but can easily be doubled or tripled for a larger group of people.

Wheat Free Crispy Large Shrimp

Crisply large shrimp make a delicious appetizer, but you may have stopped eating them since you decide to start focusing on wheat free cooking. The good news is that you can begin enjoying those delicious, crispy shrimp once again with this wonderful recipe that contains absolutely no wheat at all. These make wonderful appetizers that work well for parties. Another option is to add some sweet and sour sauce to the shrimp and serve with rice to turn this appetizer into a full, tasty meal. Just a few ingredients add up to make an awesome appetizer that is wonderful anytime.

What You'll Need:

¼ cup of wheat free flour (such as rice flour)
1 tablespoon of corn starch
2 tablespoons of baking powder
Canola oil or peanut oil for frying (do not use peanut oil if you have nut allergies)
Water
30 large shrimp that have been peeled, deveined and cooked

How to Make It:

Carefully dry the shrimp with some paper towels to ensure the batter will stick well instead of sliding off.

Mix together the baking powder, cornstarch and flour with a small amount of water to make a very thick batter. It must be thick so it does not just slide off your shrimp. Toss shrimp in the batter.

Heat oil in a skillet or in a fryer until a little batter will sizzle and cook fast.

Drop in 5-7 large shrimp into the oil, cooking until golden brown and batter is puffed and cooked well. This takes approximately 2 minutes. Use a slotted metal spoon to remove the shrimp, draining on a plate lined with paper towels. Keep the shrimp warm until you have all the shrimp fried up.

Serve as an appetizer with a nice selection of dipping sauces. Makes 30 shrimp.

Wheat Free Baked Cherry Tomatoes

These baked cherry tomatoes add a healthy appetizer to any menu. They are easy to make and can be whipped up quickly. They make a colorful addition to any appetizer table if you are hosting a party or you can simply make them for a healthy snack to be enjoyed at any time.

What You'll Need:

40 cherry tomatoes (the fresher the better)
2 tablespoons of red wine vinegar
2-4 teaspoons of olive oil

How to Make It:

Preheat oven to 400F.

Wash cherry tomatoes and dry thoroughly.

Place tomatoes on a baking dish, using a knife to slice into them to about a third of their depth. Use the sharp knife to widen the slit a bit so the drizzled oil and vinegar will seep into the tomatoes.

Drizzle with the olive oil and then drizzle the tomatoes

with the red wine vinegar, working to ensure that plenty of the vinegar goes down into the tomatoes.

Bake at 400F for about 10 minutes. Serve while warm.

Easy Wheat Free Chicken Nuggets

Chicken nuggets are a wonderful finger food that can be served up as an appetizer. Kids and adults both love these crisp, nuggets of tasty, juicy chicken. The great thing about them is that they boast a polenta coating that is wheat free, so you can stay to your wheat free diet. These little bites of flavor are much healthier for you than what you can buy at the store or at a fast food joint. They get baked, reducing the fat, and you can serve them up with many different dipping sauces for a special appetizer or a great snack.

What You'll Need:

4 boneless, skinless chicken breasts
2 large eggs, beaten
1 cup of polenta grains
1 teaspoon of herbs or seasoning (pick your favorite for chicken)

How to Make It:

Preheat the oven to 400F.

Spray a baking tray with non-stick spray. You may need a

second tray, since the nuggets must be spread out into a single layer on the trays. However, you can bake both trays at the same time as long as they fit on a single rack in the oven.

Take the chicken breasts and cut them into nugget sizes, about two inches square. Keep the sizes even for even baking.

In a large bowl, beat the egg. In a wide bowl or a large plate, mix the seasoning and polenta grains until well combined.

Drop the pieces of chicken into the bowl containing egg, making sure all the chicken is well coated with the beaten egg. A couple at a time, remove chicken pieces from the egg mixture, dipping into the polenta mix and ensuring that each piece has a nice coating. Remove and place on the baking pans. Finish the process with the rest of the chicken pieces.

Bake at 400F for about 20-25 minutes or until the chicken is cooked through, browned and crispy. To check for doneness, poke one of the largest pieces with a fork or skewer, ensuring that the juices run clear.

Serve hot with a variety of sauces. Left overs can be

saved and eaten cold as a snack, cut up into salads or added to school lunches for kids. Makes 4-6 servings.

Wheat Free Leek Tart

For an elegant occasion, this leek tart makes a delicious appetizer. Although the pastry is wheat free, it bakes up nicely, providing a crisply, flaky finish to the leeks that all your guests are sure to enjoy. You may even want to adapt this recipe and turn it into a nice main course from time to time.

What You'll Need:

Pastry Ingredients:
½ cup of gluten free flour
½ cup of brown rice flour
1 teaspoon of xanthan gum
½ cup of margarine or butter (butter preferred)
Small amount of water for mixing
Filling Ingredients:
1 tablespoon of olive oil
½ cup of boiling water
1 ½ cubes of wheat free vegetable stock
3 large eggs, well beaten
1 cup of plain, unflavored Greek yogurt
3-4 leeks, trimmed and sliced thin
Salt and pepper to taste

How to Make It:

Preheat oven to 400F.

In a medium saucepan, place olive oil and leaks, sweating them on very low heat until the leeks become soft.

Make the strong vegetable stock with the boiling water and cubs of stock, pouring the stock over the leeks and then simmering uncovered until the leeks absorb all the stock. Stir on a regular basis to avoid sticking or burning.

Meanwhile, mix together the fat, xanthan gum and flours in a medium bowl until you have a crumbly mixture. Add some water a little at a time until the mixture binds together and becomes a nice pastry dough.

Prepare a 8-9 inch flan dish with oil and flour. Press the pastry dough into the prepared dish, using hands to press it all around the sides. Do not try to use a rolling pin to roll the dough out, since it will be too fragile. Simply use your hands to cover the dish with the pastry.

Spoon leeks into the pastry shell. Mix seasonings, eggs and yogurt together, combining. Pour yogurt mixture on top of the leeks.

Bake at 400F for 35-40 minutes on the oven's middle shelf. When done, it should be firm on top and a nice, golden brown.

Allow to sit a few minutes after removing from the oven, then cutting into 10-12 small appetizer servings. You can cut into larger servings if you are using the tart for a meal.

Chapter 6: Wheat Free Breakfast Recipes

Figuring out what to eat for breakfast when you are eating wheat free can be a bit difficult. However, with a bit of work, you can find some delicious breakfast options that taste great and give you a breakfast to keep you going through the day. The following are some excellent wheat free recipes you can use for breakfast. Try a few of these recipes and have fun coming up with little adaptations that best suit you and your family. From smoked salmon breakfast to wheat free fruit salads, these recipes offer you many great options to enjoy in the mornings.

Wheat Free Smoked Salmon Egg Dish Recipe

This delicious breakfast wheat free recipe allows you to enjoy smoked salmon, which is a heart healthy protein source. Eggs add an extra protein punch to the meal. Serve up with some wheat free bagels, some oatcakes or even some seasonal fruit for a well rounded breakfast.

What You'll Need:

8 medium eggs, well beaten
1 ½ cup of smoked salmon
2-4 teaspoons of butter
4 tablespoons of milk
Salt and pepper to taste

How to Make It:

Mix beaten eggs and milk together in a bowl. Melt butter in a medium skillet. Scrambled the eggs up in the skillet until well cooked, seasoning to taste with salt and pepper. When eggs are almost done, add in strips on smoked salmon, cooking long enough to warm the salmon. Serve immediately while hot. Makes four servings.

Delicious Wheat Free Flaxseed Fruit Salad Recipe

A fruit salad makes a wonderful, healthy breakfast and the addition of flaxseed adds some healthy fats to the mix. Serve alongside a morning bagel or with a poached egg on wheat free toast for a delicious, healthy breakfast. Leftover fruit salad makes a wonderful, healthy snack you can enjoy later without guilt as well.

What You'll Need:

2 ripe bananas, chopped
3 cups of diced papaya
2 pears (any kind), peeled and chopped
2 tablespoons of rice bran
2 tablespoons of ground flaxseeds

How to Make It:

After chopping all the fruit, combine all the ingredients together, serving right away. You can also make the fruit salad the night before, cutting down on prep time in the morning and allowing the fruit to refrigerate overnight.

Wheat Free Toad in the Hole Bake Recipe

Coming up with a wheat free version of this recipe can be difficult, since the batter often ends up flattening. This recipe allows you to enjoy this breakfast again without any flatness. Enjoy the sausage version or eliminate the sausages from the recipe for a vegetarian breakfast if you wish.

What You'll Need:

¼ cup of potato starch flour
½ cup of rice flour
3 teaspoons of tapioca flour
Pinch of salt and pepper
1 tablespoon of olive oil plus ½ teaspoon of olive oil, divided
1 ½ cups of milk
8 wheat free sausages
2 eggs, well beaten

How to Make It:

Mix together the milk, flours, pepper, salt and eggs in a large mixing bowl. Beat the ingredients together with a whisk until bubbly. Another option is to use a blender or food processor to make the batter. Once combined, but the batter in the refrigerator for 30 minutes.

Preheat the oven to 400F.

10 minutes before the batter needs to come out of the fridge, place 1 tablespoon of the olive oil into a 11x9 inch glass or metal baking dish, placing into the oven to heat up the olive oil.

Meanwhile, add the ½ teaspoon of olive oil to a skillet, browning the sausages in the oil, making sure that the skins are well browned. You do not need to cook the sausages all the way through at this time. Remove the baking dish from the oven, carefully putting the sausages into the hot oil, avoiding any splashes. Place the baking dish with the sausages back into the oven, allowing the oil to get hot again.

Take the batter from the fridge, giving it another quick beating. Pull the sausages from the oven, pouring the egg batter over top of the sausages. It is important that the oil is very hot and the batter should sizzle when poured over the hot oil. This helps to give your dish crisp edge and a crisp bottom.

Place the baking dish back in the oven, baking at 400F

for 30 minutes. Remove from the oven, serving while it is hot. It should be soft inside and nice and crispy outside, offering a delicious, warm breakfast. Makes 4 servings.

Gluten Free 1-Person Breakfast Omelet

If you need a quick breakfast dish for just one person, this 1-person omelet is an easy breakfast to whip up. It combines some delicious vegetables with the eggs for a healthy omelet. You can try different variations of this recipe by simply changing the vegetables added to the omelet or by topping with different types of cheese.

What You'll Need:

1 tablespoon of milk
2 eggs, beaten
1 tablespoon of celery, finely chopped
1 tablespoon of chives, finely chopped
1 tablespoon of leeks, finely chopped
Salt and pepper to taste
¼ cup of grated mozzarella cheese, plus extra cheese for topping

How to Make It:

Combine together all ingredients (except extra cheese for topping). Mix ingredients together into well combined.

In a frying pan or skillet, melt butter or use cooking spray to prepare the pan. When pan is hot, pour the egg mixture into the pan. Cook on low heat, raising the omelet from time to time to allow the uncooked eggs run down into the frying pan. When well cooked, fold over to finish cooking, sprinkling with a small amount of cheese. Place on a plate, topping with some extra chives as a nice garnish.

Add mushrooms, onions, bacon, tomato, green peppers or other vegetables for delicious, healthy variations of this one-person omelet.

Wheat Free Blueberry Breakfast Muffins Recipe

If you miss eating delicious breakfast muffins, you are sure to love this delicious muffin recipe, which is completely wheat free. You will need a gluten free self raising flour, which is fairly easy to find. Try shopping for it online if you cannot find it at your local stores. The fruit contained in the muffins add extra servings of fruit to your day. You can even freeze extra muffins and pop them out for a delicious breakfast treat any time. Make a double batch if you want to have plenty to throw in the freezer for later.

What You'll Need:

1 egg
2 tablespoons of canola oil
1 cup of skim milk
2 ½ cups of gluten free self raising flour
¼ cup of sugar
1 cup of frozen blueberries
How to Make It:
Preheat oven to 325F.

In a large bowl, combine together the sugar and flour. In

a smaller bowl, combine the milk, oil and egg, mixing well. Add wet ingredients to the dry ingredients, mixing well until thoroughly combined. Fold in the cup of frozen blueberries, stirring to distribute berries throughout the batter.

Grease a muffin tray or line the muffin tin with liners. Pour batter into muffin tin, filling each one about ¾ of the way full. Bake for about 15-20 minutes on 325 until golden brown on top. Enjoy eating them while they are warm and freeze any leftovers to keep them fresh.

You can change this recipe just a bit to enjoy different flavors of muffins. Add in any other berries, instead of blueberries. You can also add in a couple mashed bananas instead of the berries for banana muffins. A cup of stewed apples can be added for delicious apple breakfast muffins.

Chapter 7: Wheat Free Dessert Recipes

Just because you are focusing on wheat free cooking does not mean that you have to give up desserts. You can make a variety of delectable desserts without using wheat products. From simple desserts like baked bananas to an elegant chocolate soufflé, here are some wonderful wheat free recipes you can use to create amazing desserts that will not make you feel deprived at all.

Wheat Free Baked Nutty Bananas

These delicious bananas are fully of nutty, sweet goodness and make a wonderful dessert after dinner or a warm evening snack to enjoy. With minimal sugar, this dessert is a healthy choice that will help you eliminate your sweet cravings with a wholesome dessert.

What You'll Need:

4 large, firm bananas
4 tablespoons of pecans, chopped
2 tablespoons of soft, dark brown sugar
Honey for drizzling

How to Make It:

Preheat the oven to 350F.

On a baking sheet, place the bananas an equal distance apart. Bananas should be left in their skins. Bake at 350 for 20-30 minutes. The peel will be black when they are done.

Remove bananas from the oven, removing the bananas from the skins very carefully, since hot banana can quickly cause bad burns. Place each banana on a separate dish or in a separate bowl. Slice into pieces with a knife.

Sprinkle the bananas with brown sugar and chopped pecans. Allow the bananas to sit for 3-4 minutes to allow the sugar to begin melting. Top with just a drizzle of honey and then serve while warm. You can even serve over ice cream or top the bananas with a small amount of whipped cream to add something extra to the delicious dessert.

Wheat Free Pumpkin Pie

Pumpkin is very good for you, since it is high in fiber and a great source of vitamin A. It can quickly be turned into a wonderful dessert, even if you are cooking without wheat. This wheat free recipe uses a crust made from wheat free ingredients. While you can use fresh pumpkin, if you do use canned pumpkin, make sure the pumpkin you purchase is pure pumpkin so you avoid any added ingredients. This makes a great fall dessert, but it tastes great all year round with a bit of whipped cream on top.

What You'll Need:

Pie Crust Ingredients:

1/3 cup of gluten free flour
½ cup of sweet white rice flour
3 tablespoons of sugar
1 large egg yolk
1 teaspoon of xanthan gum
1 tablespoon of water
½ cup of butter, softened (and a little additional butter to butter the pie dish)
Filling Ingredients:

¼ cup of sugar

1 cup of pumpkin (mashed if using fresh pumpkin)

1 large egg, well beaten

¾ cup of evaporated milk

½ teaspoon of pumpkin pie spice

How to Make It:

Preheat oven to 425F.

Take an 8 inch pie dish and butter it lightly, then dusting it with a bit of rice flour. Place the pie dish on a larger baking sheet to avoid spills when baking.

Place softened butter, sugar, flours and xanthan gum in a large mixing bowl, mixing well until you have a crumbly mixture. Add in the water and the egg yolk, mixing and kneading until you have a nice ball of pastry dough. Add a bit more water if the dough is still crumbly and dry.

Once you have a smooth ball of dough, lightly flour a surface and then roll out the pastry dough until it is large enough to line the pie dish. Press into the pie dish, trimming the edges. For dough that is too fragile, simply press the pastry dough right into the pie dish with floured hands, trimming the edges when done if you need to.

For the filling, combined spices and sugar in a mixing bowl, combining well. Add in pumpkin, mixing well. Then, add the beaten egg, mixing thoroughly. Last, stir in evaporated milk, mixing until the batter is smooth and well combined.

Pour batter into the pie crust, filling it to the top. Once filled, place the pie in the oven, baking for 15 minutes at 425F. Reduce the oven temperature to 350F, baking the pie for another 30-40 minutes.

To check for doneness, check after about 25 minutes at 350F, using a fork, toothpick or thin knife right into the pie's center. Continue baking if the pie is still runny. If the filling is completely set in the center, you can remove the pie from the oven.

Allow pie to cool in the pie dish, serving at room temperature or refrigerate the pie and serve it cold. Make sure the pie is stored in a refrigerator to keep in from going bad. When serving, top with fresh whipped cream or a small amount of vanilla ice cream. Makes 8 servings.

Wheat Free Chocolate Soufflé

This elegant dessert is perfect for an elegant dinner party and it tastes so amazing, no one will know that it is both wheat free and gluten free. To ensure you get the rich, chocolate flavor, go with dark chocolate that uses at least 70% cacao in it. Quality cocoa powder is important as well. For the dark chocolate, Green & Black's organic chocolate is a perfect choice. This recipe makes four servings, so you may need to double it if you are making the dessert for a larger crowd.

What You'll Need:

5 teaspoons of unsweetened cocoa powder
1 tablespoon of wheat free flour
4 medium eggs, separated
¼ cup of light brown sugar
6 tablespoons of double cream (heavy cream)
¾ cup of grated dark chocolate, melted
Pinch of cream of tarter
Several drops of vanilla
Small amount of butter to grease ramekins or soufflé dish
¼ powdered sugar

How to Make It:

Preheat oven to 375F.

Use butter to lightly butter 4 large ramekins or a large 1 liter soufflé dish.

In a medium saucepan, add flour, sugar and cocoa powder, adding in the cream gradually while beating until you have a smooth mixture. Turn on low heat under the pan, stirring continuously until the sugar melts. Stirring is important to avoid burning or overheating the sugar.

Remove saucepan from heat, adding in egg yolks, one yolk at a time, beating each one well with the mixture before adding the next yolk. Next, add in the vanilla and melted chocolate, mixing well until thoroughly combined.

In a large, clean bowl, beat egg whites until they begin forming peaks. Add in the pinch of cream of tartar, continuing to whisk eggs until the cream of tartar is well mixed into the egg whites. Gently fold egg whites into the chocolate mixture. Do so a single spoonful at a time so you avoid eliminating the air you have beaten into the whipped egg whites.

Spoon the chocolate mixture into the ramekins or the large soufflé dish. If using ramekins, place on a baking tray to make it easier to move in and out of the oven. Bake for 30 minutes at 375 and do not open the oven door while the soufflé is baking.

When fully cooked, the soufflé should look firm on top and should have risen well. Serve while hot, topped with a bit of sifted powdered sugar. It should be eaten while warm, since it does not keep well after it cools.

Wheat Free Apple Cake Recipe

Delicious apples with a nice, moist cake make a wonderful dessert, especially when this cake is warm. The cake tastes amazing and it is not overly sweet.

What You'll Need:

1/3 cup of sugar
2/3 cup of rice flour
¼ cup of butter
1/3 cup of soy flour
1 egg
¼ cup of milk
2 teaspoons of baking powder
1 lemon, juiced
½ teaspoon of vanilla
3 medium granny smith apples, peeled, cored and thinly sliced
Extra sugar and cinnamon for sprinkling

How to Make It:

Preheat the oven to 350F.

Use a bit of butter or cooking spray to grease a 8 inch

round cake pan.

In a large mixing bowl, cream sugar and butter together. Add in the egg, beating well to combined.

In another bowl, sift together baking powder and flours.

Add half of the dry mixture to the wet mixture, beating until combined. Add in some of the milk. Add the rest of the flour mixture, beating again, then adding the rest of the milk. Continue to beat mixture until all ingredients are well combined.

Spread cake batter into the round cake pan, smoothing out the top.

Once the apples have been peeled, cored and sliced thinly, squeeze the lemon juice over them to keep them from getting brown and to add some flavor. Arrange the apple slices on top of the cake batter.

Place in the oven, baking for an hour at 350F. The apples should be golden brown on top and the cake should be cooked all the way through.

Remove from the oven, sprinkling the top of the cake with cinnamon and sugar while it is still hot. Serve warm with small scoops of ice cream. Makes 8 servings.

Wheat Free Double Chocolate Chip Cookies

Indulge in your chocolate cravings with these double chocolate chip cookies. They use rice flour, so they are completely wheat free. If you have nut allergies as well, make sure you check the chocolate chips to ensure they are made in a nut free environment.

What You'll Need:

1/4 cup of granulated sugar
½ cup of butter
1/3 cup of brown sugar
½ teaspoon of vanilla
1 medium egg, well beaten
2 tablespoons of unsweetened cocoa powder
½ teaspoon of baking soda
2 teaspoons of instant coffee granules
½ teaspoon of baking powder
¾ cup of rice flour
2/3 cup of chocolate chips of chunks
How to Make It:
Preheat oven to 350F.

Line cookie sheets with parchment paper or other non-stick baking paper.

Place sugars and butter in a large bowl, beating to cream together until very smooth. Beat in the vanilla and egg slowly.

In another bowl, combine together all the dry ingredients. Pour dry ingredients into the wet ingredients, mixing together to combine. Last, add in the chocolate chips, stirring until chocolate chips are well distributed throughout the cookie dough.

Drop teaspoonfuls of cookie dough onto the prepared cookie sheets. Space out the cookies evenly, since the dough will spread a bit during the baking process.

Bake cookies for 12-13 minutes. Cookies should be firm to touch when they are done.

Allow cookies to cool a few minutes on the cookie sheets, then place on a baking rack to allow them to completely cool. Once cool, store cookies in an airtight container to keep them fresh. Cookies taste delicious both warm and cold and will keep for 2-4 days.

Makes about 40 cookies.

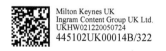